INTRODUCTION:

How does hypnosis work? Would you like to learn hypnosis? Maybe you're interested in hypnosis, or maybe you want to become a hypnotherapist. Whether you want to become a hypnotist or just want to learn it for yourself, this book will hold the key to learning the key component of hypnosis and help you use it to take back control of your life! As a practicing hypnotherapist of years, I've been a little bit disheartened with the way hypnosis is presented in the media, by social media, and unfortunately by many hypnotists as well. Many people use terminology that doesn't really make any practical sense, and confuses people! Hypnosis transforms lives! Whether you want to learn clinical hypnosis, stage hypnosis, comedy hypnosis, or anything else, I hope this book serves as a guide to help you learn it in a simple, easy-to-understand way that anyone can pick up and appreciate!

(NOTE: This book is not intended to be a substitute for professional medical advice, diagnosis, or treatment. Always seek the advice of your physician or other qualified health provider with any questions you may have regarding a medical condition. Never disregard professional medical advice.)

CHAPTER ONE:
WHAT IS HYPNOSIS?

What does it mean to be hypnotized? WHAT is hypnosis? Hypnosis is FOCUS! FOCUS which puts you in a trance. Generally, "hypnosis" and "trance" mean the same thing. You go into hypnosis many times a day! All you need to do to enter a trance is to put your focus on something. That's why many hypnotists induct their clients by having them stare at a ceiling (the most common induction I personally use) because it captures their FOCUS. Daydreaming, brainstorming, texting, calling, having a conversation, even EMOTIONS can count as trances. Why? Because, they capture your FOCUS! So, hypnosis is a focused trance which can make positive changes or affect behavior. It's sort of like opening the door to your subconscious. A light trance might let you just stick your hand in, a moderate trance might let you peek your head in, and a deep enough trance will let you walk into the room. The programming for many behaviors is held in the subconscious mind, so in many cases hypnosis is at least partially necessary for someone to resolve a problem. But, why does hypnosis 'open the door' to the subconscious? Why does it have this effect? The reason is actually very simple! It has to do with our brain waves. There are three brainwaves associated with hypnosis. And, by 'brainwave' I'm talking about the speed at which your brain fires information. Hypnotic trances (unless you're doing an instant induction, which I will get into later) use focus and relaxation to slow down your brainwaves to the ALPHA brainwave or lower! THAT is why hypnosis has the ability to 'open the door' to the subconscious. Your subconscious becomes more and more open to suggestion depending on how low of a brainwave your brain is operating. I want to clarify, you do NOT always need to be relaxed to be hypnotized! And honestly, if you are a hypnotist worth your salt, you are going to be able to adapt the induction to suit your client's personality (more on this later). Most hypnosis occurs at the ALPHA brainwave, but there are two below that (THETA, then DELTA). This is why hypnosis 'opens the door' to your subconscious. It's a trance which lowers your brainwave deep enough to access and make changes to the subconscious. The hypnosis brainwave is the key to accessing more ability out of your subconscious or making changes to your habits and behaviors. The change in brainwave is the KEY to accessing your mind's potential. This might sound really technical, but really hypnosis feels AMAZING. When you come out of hypnosis it can feel like you just had the world's best power nap. Also, the more you do hypnosis (whether self-hypnosis or hypnosis by someone else), the MORE easy it is to go deeper the next time! And, let's clear this out of the way... NO ONE can hypnotize you to do anything you don't want to do! You are ALWAYS in control during every session!

CHAPTER TWO:
THE SUBCONSCIOUS MIND

Hypnosis is a trance which grants someone access to their subconscious mind. But, what is the subconscious mind? The subconscious mind is the part of our mind that is automatic and below the surface. In a computer there is both hardware and software. The software tells the hardware how to work. Imagine a computer with all its pieces but no code to tell it how to function. You would power it on but nothing would show up on the screen. If there are no programs then the computer doesn't know how to use its parts. Your body has hardware (your brain and body) but without the software (your subconscious mind) how will it use its parts? All you do is think "I will lift my finger", but you don't specify all the particular muscles that need to activate for the finger to move. The SUBCONSCIOUS has the 'programs' which automatically maintain the functions of your brain and body. And, sometimes those programs need correction which is done by hypnosis. Aside from the programs that maintain your bodily functions you also have MENTAL programs. There is a 'money program' which tells you whether you are rich or poor. There is the 'relationships program' which manifests good or bad relationships. There can also be a 'smoking program' which is present in people who are hooked on smoking. To change the urges, you have to change the program in the subconscious. To change the program, you use hypnosis to change the subconscious. It can be like changing the code of a program on a computer. Once it's saved, the next time the subconscious runs the program it uses a different set of instructions. The subconscious can also be used as a tool! Many influential people have used it for success. Nikola Tesla used self-hypnosis to visualize his inventions. He would visualize an idea for a machine, and his subconscious would explain every step of how to create the machine down to the angle of the screws! Mark Twain used a hypnotic technique called 'Automatic Writing' to create his stories. Nobody knows the limits of what the subconscious can accomplish, but it tends to respond to the limitations you place on yourself. When you believe "I can do this!" it says "Okay!". When you say "I can't do this!" it says "Okay!". The things that you believe about yourself are accepted by the subconscious fully. The subconscious is extremely literal, and takes things at face value. If you said "I am mad." you probably mean angry. But, the subconscious would take it as "I am insane". It does not distinguish jokes, sarcasm, or lies and takes everything literally. What most people don't realize is that THAT is why there is both a conscious and subconscious mind. The conscious mind is the wheel, and subconscious is the ship. All the mechanisms of the ship obey the steering wheel (you) but you need to learn to steer it correctly! But, most people don't even realize that they have that level of control over that steering wheel so they let it just move however it gravitates. They say "I guess the ship is just moving to the left and there's nothing I can do about it. It's just how I'm born." but that's not true! YOU are in control! Hypnosis lets you take control of that wheel and move the ship however you want! I also want to add that meditation is similar. The difference between self-hypnosis and meditation is mainly just what you do with your mind in the state of hypnosis. Self-hypnosis is you entering the state of hypnosis to tell your subconscious a message whereas meditation is you entering the state of hypnosis and letting your thoughts flow freely with no specific purpose, like your subconscious gets to tell YOU a message. Meditation is extremely useful and you should do it everyday. You don't have to do any specific cross-legged position for it to work all you need to do is sit or lay down, relax and let your mind think what it wants. The deeper you go into it the more connected you will feel to your inner mind. I honestly have no clue why people over-complicate hypnosis and meditation. It's very simple, useful and everyone alive can benefit from it. There are actually entire societies that have used it in place of modern technology (More on that later)! I'm not trying to harp on other hypnotists too much since I am by no means the only voice on this subject but the way a lot of people try to explain it is extremely obscure and makes almost zero practical sense to a non-hypnotist. "Altered state of consciousness!" What is that even trying to say?! "Altered" how? It's really like a state of awareness that EMPOWERS you to have more control over your mind. Your subconscious is about 90% more powerful than you conscious mind, holds every single memory you ever experienced, manages your brain and body, and has a collection of tools that many people are not aware they have at their disposal. The best way of looking at hypnotherapy is that you're not 'broken' needing to be fixed. Look at it like your mind is very powerful, and has a collection of amazing tools at your disposal. When you misuse the tools it can be problematic. Hypnosis is about re-framing tools, not curing problems. If you look at an issue as a 'problem' you are giving the order for it to be a problem. Is it a weight holding you down? Or, an amazing tool being used in the wrong direction? I'll give an example! One client of mine was a woman who was going to be married a few months after she asked for my help. Every-time she would practice the father-daughter dance with her father she would bawl her eyes out. She wanted to be hypnotized to not cry and ruin her makeup on her wedding day. The trigger that made her cry specifically was a song that was going to be played during the dance because it had to do with the father of a bride, and her bridesmaid recently lost her father, making even more of an emotional event. A lot of hypnotists would just hypnotize her to feel non-emotional about it. But, that's the wrong approach! Remember how I told you earlier that emotions can also be trances? Hypnosis is a trance that can affect a person's behavior. So, what was actually happening was that the song was putting her in a trance (focus) and crying was technically a hypnotic phenomena (behavior). The solution would not be to treat it as a problem that needed to be fixed but to empower her to feel more in control over the tools that are a part of her. I put her in a trance, and had her visualize the dance with her father. Then I told her "As you hear the song play now, and you notice your bridesmaid watching from across the room. You feel the emotions you were feeling before. But you now realize that there's nothing wrong with how you feel. In fact, I don't want you to stop feeling the way you do but instead you realize that the crying is not necessarily the same as having an emotion. And, as you watch yourself do this dance with your father and feel this emotion. The emotions themselves serve as an indicator that you have control over the reactions. Especially the reaction of crying. And, if you can experience that emotion it has to mean that you can do whatever you want with it. It's your emotion right? And every time you feel that emotion you feel in absolute control over your reaction over it. You can do whatever you want with it. And, if you feel that emotion as you see your bridesmaid and do your dance then surely you always have an absolute sense of control over the reaction. To the point where you even feel relaxed being this emotional. Instead of fighting this emotion, you embrace it fully as it's a tool you have control over and yours to do whatever you want with.". After two sessions, she had a pleasant experience doing that dance with zero tears shed. I like to see hypnosis work for my clients! I won't pretend that I don't want to make money from my business because I do, but seeing that what I do genuinely helps people is worth more to me than that! I also want to note! All hypnosis sessions are confidential! That story was only shared with the explicit consent of that client. Should you ever do a hypnosis session with me, the details of your session will NOT be shared publicly unless you have given consent. Let's give another example: A man wanted to stop smoking cigars and weed joints. Here's the truth about smoking addictions, it's almost never the smoking that's the problem. This particular person told me he felt nervous energy that he didn't know how to deal with so he used cigars to relax it. Typically, he would've been hypnotized to feel disgusted by the smell and taste of the cigars and joints to quit this habit. But, was his problem the cigars and joints? Or, was it his nervous energy? His nervous energy was the 'tool' within his mind that was misdirected. I did not approach him saying "Oh yes, you're so addicted to cigars, you need to be hypnotized to quit or your health will suffer and you will die.". Instead, I focused on transforming that nervous energy into positive energy so that whenever he felt the 'trigger' that would usually make him want to smoke it now made him extremely motivated and energized! He wasn't 'broken' at all! He just needed to redirect how he was using the tool that was already within his mind. After all, excitement and nervousness are basically the same reaction in the body and can be transformed relatively simply depending on how you view it. Most of the time, these 'issues' are just misused tools and if you are a hypnotist your job is to REFRAME them NOT to 'fix' something that isn't broken. There are many ways to communicate with the subconscious mind. Actually, I've seen situations where a client was under hypnosis and his subconscious mind started to speak to me as if it was a person! This person was being hypnotized for a confidence issue where he had trouble feeling like he could accomplish what he wanted. When he was under, his eyes opened at me and he said "Excuse me, sorry to bother you. I'm speaking from the subconscious level of his mind. The reason Jake has trouble with this is because he is expecting all the results immediately. He's developed apathy because when it hasn't worked the first time he gives up. That's why he has this issue.". I had a full on conversation with his subconscious mind where it told me every reason that he was having this trouble and what he needed to resolve it. "You need to teach him to be more consistent and stick to his plans. Empower him to live a better life.". "Is there anything else I need to tell him?" I asked. "No, that's it. Thank you.". I then woke him up from his trance and he was in total shock of what just happened. The subconscious will listen to what you tell it SPECIFICALLY. Although this person's mind did it on it's own, you have to SPECIFY what you want it to do. If you speak to it as if it's purely robotic, it can respond with robotic like mannerisms (Yes, No, I don't know) but if you specify that it will communicate in a specific way it can respond back to that specific instruction. "You will now speak to me verbally.". This is extremely useful in finding out why people have the troubles that they do. Like I said, the subconscious has access to all your memories and is able to tell you why something is acting the way it is. The subconscious won't lie unless the client wants to lie. Even forensic hypnotists cannot force the truth out of someone. Anytime you are hypnotized you are in 100% control. Even if you feel that your mind is blank or hazy your subconscious will reject any and all bad suggestions, or things said to you that you do not want to have happen. So, you cannot force anyone to say anything they don't want to and you cannot force someone to quit smoking. People will only do what they want. You can't imagine how pissed the hypnotist community gets when movies create evil hypnotist characters that mind control their subjects. That does NOT work and even if someone tried it, it would fail. The subconscious is a force only for your good. What you also need to understand is that sometimes people's 'problems' might not even be 'misused tools' but an attempt by someone's mind to grow. Basically, growing pains. As if their mind was like a plant with its roots extending down the soil and hitting a rock. And, let's be honest! You can't expect everyone to relax! Say someone was being hypnotized for post traumatic stress disorder (assuming that's legal in your state, province, and or country). How do you get them into trance? Don't try to stop how they feel. Re-frame it to their advantage! What if they can't focus because they feel nervous? Or, they have a horrible attention span? That's where you MATCH their emotions (which is what qualifies as their trance) and cater suggestions towards their current feeling. Example: "I'm glad you knew you needed to feel nervous to be hypnotized. You can let yourself feel nervous. In fact, don't let that feeling go for another ten seconds...". Both positive AND negative emotions can put a person into a trance. I have known hypnotists who turned people away because they were nervous and couldn't focus. The key is to re-frame is so that the negative emotion (which counts as an emotional trance) is what pushes them TOWARDS their goal. "That's right. It's okay to be nervous. In fact, that feeling you have right now only allows you to focus more on the sound of my voice as you hold it for as long as you need. And, if you want to hold onto it for now as you focus only on the sound of my voice, that's okay. Or, if you want you can let it go as you relax deeper and focus just on the sound of my voice feeling more relaxed by the second...". It's also helpful to let people choose what they want to do. There are two main paths with hypnosis. DIRECT and INDIRECT! Direct hypnosis is "You see the door in front of you as you relax now. You walk up to it, open the door and walk inside.".Indirect hypnosis is like saying "You see multiple doors in front of you... what do they look like? All of them lead to your desired outcome... I wonder which door you choose to take now as you walk up to it and open it." Some people are very heavy on only one path of hypnosis, becoming only a direct or indirect hypnotist. Honestly, you want to be able to draw from both. Some people respond better to direct, others indirect, or you could use a mix of both depending on the client's personality. Don't overthink it! The key is let them decide how things look to them. For example: I don't say "Imagine yourself holding a red balloon". It's better to let their subconscious decide the color and imagery. "Imagine yourself holding a balloon. What hand are you holding it in? What color is it? How long is the string?". The reason for this is that if you try to specify every detail it may conflict with how your client intuitively thinks of it. If you say "You see a sandy beach with golden sand beneath your feet." and your client is thinking of white sand instead, then it can conflict with the process. This is really good for people who are skeptical and have control issues. Instead of going through the door that I say, they can pick from one of three potential doors (and all of them lead to the same place). Typically, the more you want hypnosis to work, the quicker you can go into a trance. This is not the sort of thing where you wanting for it makes you needy or desperate. Actually, the most responsive clients I have had are usually the ones desperate for it to work. Also, DO NOT become a 'follower' of any one person. You should instead learn from as many hypnotists as possible and develop your own style of doing it. The hypnosis that I do is called "Ericksonian (Indirect) Hypnosis". Yes, Milton Erickson was an amazing hypnotist. NO, I don't think he was always right or was the 'best' hypnotist because there is no 'best' way to do hypnosis there is only YOUR best. Maybe your thing is direct hypnosis, maybe it's more indirect. Maybe it's conversational hypnosis. Or, maybe you're the best at storytelling and that's how you do your trances. Maybe you forgo all of that and prefer to do stage and comedy hypnosis. You have to test the waters with different styles and create your own! ANY hypnotist who claims they know the 'best' way to do it is a fraud, and should not be taken seriously.

CHAPTER THREE: TRANCES

We've already established that trances are what you put your focus on. There are many kinds of trances, and there are different indicators that someone is in a trance. One of the most overlooked, however, are EMOTIONAL trances. EMOTIONS can put you into a trance because they sustain your focus. Anger, depression, anxiety, fear, hate, love, joy, and really any emotion you hold onto for a sustained period of time can put you into a trance. There are all sorts of trances for all sorts of behaviors. In one book, there was a story of a psychiatrist and hypnotist who was working in a hospital. A woman was taken in on a stretcher who was having an absolute meltdown. Swearing, kicking, and screaming. The hospital staff apologized and said "We're sorry, this woman is schizophrenic." He walked up closer, observed how she was acting, and said "She's not schizophrenic." This surprised the hospital staff. "What do you mean?" they replied. "She's in an age-regressed trance. She's having a temper tantrum like a child." The woman was in a trance which caused her to act like, and have the mannerisms of, a child. She wasn't schizophrenic but had severe personality issues. The point is that a LOT of issues can seem like they are a mental issue when they are in reality just trances people don't know that they're in. Remember, I said a trance is focus which can AFFECT or CAUSE behavior. The focus was maybe some event or experience she went through as a child, and the behavior was the result of that focus, creating an emotional hypnosis. A LOT of issues get misdiagnosed because doctors, psychologists, and psychiatrists generally don't know that much about hypnosis in the west. This does not mean that doctors and therapists are intending to lie; they're usually just misinformed. It doesn't help that media and fake performances create a false representation of what hypnosis is, so it can ward them off from wanting to learn more about it. I believe that in Eastern Europe, it's more common for psychiatrists to use hypnosis, but unfortunately, in the west, it hasn't really caught up. Many doctors and therapists unknowingly put their clients into trances without knowing it. If they ask their client or patient to recall a memory with vivid details, that focus puts them into a trance. This can make the words of the therapist or doctor act as suggestions to the subconscious, which may actually do more harm than help unless they change the memory in some way. Otherwise, they'd just be reinforcing the memory as negative. Like I said before, there are different kinds of trances. Actually, most of what you do as a hypnotist is taking them out of a trance instead of putting them in one. A lot of what we call mental "issues" are just trances people don't know they're in. Insomnia is a trance. Overthinking is a trance. PTSD could be considered a trance (The triggers are the focus, panic attacks are the behavior). Like I said, a trance is focus which affects or causes a behavior. There are both positive and negative trances, and you need to consider whether it's worth creating a new trance or simply removing the old one. People's life situations can also count as trances. In your subconscious, you are programmed to be either poor, middle class, or wealthy. If someone's mind is set to be poor and they try to become wealthy without changing what is in the subconscious, it's like trying to walk past a brick wall. Their financial status is the trance that they're in. Someone might constantly end up in bad relationships because they're in a trance that tells them they don't deserve anything better. Pretty much your entire life is made up of trances, and you have to decide what kind you will allow into it! I've also noticed that there are 'mini trances' people enter for a really short period of time. These trances don't really do much, but you can see someone's mannerisms change for a brief period of time. Play someone's favorite childhood song and watch their face fill with the excitement of that 10-year-old kid they used to be when they listened to it. Watch them light up with the same child-like excitement they had at that age. That's an age-regressive trance. The focus is the music, the behavior is the body language and mannerisms that they feel. One big example of this (that NOBODY is talking about) is autism. A lot of people who are in a heavy age-regressive trance are mistaken for autistic. It's usually that someone is abused/neglected heavily as a child, which causes a part of their mind to be partially stuck as a child, which causes them to have a difficult time understanding social cues and take things very literally. You can actually age regress people with hypnosis. This can be for the sake of processing emotions, recalling memories, or as a stage trick. This is a kind of emotional trance, and is usually done as a way of coping with a traumatic event. I am NOT saying that autism is not real (it definitely is). But, if you think about it logically, there are so many examples where someone is sexually abused at a very young age, then they hold onto child-like mannerisms and behaviors (which includes not understanding social cues) because a part of them is stuck at that age, and then they're diagnosed with "Autism". That is not autism, that is age regression. The real issue should be very obvious. Another overlooked trance is music. Michael Jackson used special patterns in his music that would quickly put people into trances. This was to absorb people in the world of his songs. Basically, what he did was make all the sound effects and instruments "bounce" off of each other in a way that was harmonious. That way, you would constantly be hearing different sounds that were of the same pattern, which would put you into a quick trance and absorb you into the world of the song. There are many kinds of trances, and you enter them every day. So, how do you use trances to your benefit with hypnosis? There is a general pattern of using trances when it comes to hypnotherapy. It usually goes as follows: Induction, Deepener, Safe-Place, Suggestions, Post-Hypnotic Suggestions, Forward-Pacing, and Anchors.

An induction is to get them to relax and get their subconscious to focus on your suggestions. Deepener is to deepen the amount of relaxation and bring them to a closer state of hypnosis (Relaxation to the point of the Alpha brainwave). Safe-place means mentally immersing them in a place where they feel safe and relaxed. It's better to let them decide what their safe-place looks like. You do this by having them take notes. "Notice the temperature of this place, how does it smell? What does the ground look like? Sand? Dirt? Gravel? Rocks? Are there any small animals walking around? Are you alone, or surrounded by people who care about you?" I'm not saying the hypnosis won't work if you tell them what it looks like, but maybe you said "You are walking across a sandy beach. You look down and see the white sand as it envelopes your feet." and THEY are thinking of it like a hiking trail where they're wearing steel-toe boots. Use hypnosis scripts as a helper but don't go word for word. One client I had was an elderly woman who was AFRAID of forests. I (as a new hypnotist) used a FOREST safe-place for her session. Her session (pain relief hypnosis) did not work as well because of the imagery I used for her, and she requested a different kind after the session was over. Learn from my mistake. Now, there's suggestions. There are MANY ways to do suggestions, just like there are many ways to do hypnosis. In general, you'll use some form of imagery that has to do with their issue or goal. But, it's very important to know when to be direct or indirect with your suggestions. Example: One client I had was a person who had trouble visualizing. He wanted to be hypnotized to be better at visualizing so he could be better at meditating. I had him under hypnosis, then told him "In this room, you see your imagination in the form of a camera, you pick it up. What does it look like?" "It's old, dirty, it's not working," he said back. "Why do you think so?" I asked him. "I don't know, it's just not working," he replied. I had him visualize that camera projecting an image onto the screen, which he described as grainy and scratchy. After that, I had him imagine that his old camera was now upgraded to a brand new, modern, highest-end camera capable of producing new films in the highest resolutions. This new camera also had the ability to fill in any details for any image it captures, so that he didn't even need to specify it himself. I then had him visualize that brand new camera projecting a film onto the screen. I said "How does it look now?" He said "It's a much better picture, the quality is better." At the end of the session, I had him visualize him using his brand new camera one more time, and he had much better results with his meditation. This is an example of both DIRECT and INDIRECT hypnosis. I was direct in that I told him he would see a camera, but I was indirect in that I let his subconscious decide what the camera would look like. How would it have gone if I told him "You now see a rusty, broken old camera." and he was imagining a working one? Be direct in the direction you are going with your session but be careful not to let your own ego interfere with the actual issue at hand. Post-hypnotic suggestions are suggestions you want to include to lock in the suggestions you just made. If one of your suggestions was "You hate cigarettes." then a good post-hypnotic suggestion is "Every time you see a cigarette, you feel disgusted." or "Every time you hold a cigarette, you feel an overwhelming urge to throw it in the garbage". You can change this for whatever your goal is. Forward-pacing is important because it can reinforce the specific goal that you or your client has. If you gave someone suggestions and post-hypnotic suggestions for quitting smoking, then forward-pacing is having them imagine the future where their goal is already achieved. They'd probably be visualizing the entire time, but this kind of visualization locks in that their desired goal has presently happened. The subconscious only knows the present, not the past or future. That is part of why memories from years ago can make you feel horrible today. Anytime the memory is played, it's taken as if it's the current future. So, forward-pacing takes all the suggestions you just gave and makes it the PRESENT! So, if you're trying to do stop smoking hypnosis, this part makes it that they have already quit smoking, not that they will in the future; otherwise, they will always be ABOUT to quit smoking but never there. After forward-pacing, you can use Anchors. Anchors aren't always necessary, but there usually is no reason not to use them. They're a special type of post-hypnotic suggestion that reinforces positive feelings. Say someone got stressed during their work meetings. You could say "Every time you rub your thumb, you feel immediately relaxed." Whether to use Anchors or not is at your discretion, but they're especially useful for anxiety-type issues. And, don't feel like you have to follow this EXACT order anytime you hypnotize yourself or a client. You can use your own discretion to judge what is best for each person. There was one person (who I did pain relief for) who I did do post-hypnotic suggestions and forward-pacing for but not anchors since he didn't need it in his case. That had no effect on how well his hypnosis worked, and by the end of it, he told me that his legs "felt like they had springs in them". The thing to remember is that you don't have to be boring with hypnosis. Have fun with it!

CHAPTER FOUR: INDUCTIONS

How do you do an induction? There are many kinds of inductions. There are progressive, rapid, and instant inductions. Progressive and rapid inductions work by relaxing the client, and instant inductions work through pattern interruption. Relaxation helps to relax and reprogram the pre-frontal cortex (thinking brain). When hypnotized, you might actually notice a fuzzy or hazy feeling in your forehead. That is the pre-frontal cortex relaxing. The difference between progressive and rapid inductions is very simple. Progressive is you relaxing progressively (usually like 10-15 minutes for this induction), and rapid inductions are you relaxing quickly (under a few minutes). In a lot of cases the bad "instructions" are held in the pre-frontal cortex, relaxing it (with hypnosis) allows it to be reprogrammed (it's not the pre-frontal cortex 100% of the time). In a brain of someone with PTSD, doctors can see changes in the activity between the amygdala (fear, stress response) and hippocampus (memory). But, why would that be? You're basically bypassing the re-frontal cortex. Because, it's the pre-frontal cortex that gives the direction to those other two parts. Basically, the brain doesn't have a "hardware" problem it has a "software" problem. The changes in the brain are a reflection of the "software" (the wiring of your brain is your THOUGHTS). When you hypnotize someone, you're changing the directions given to the brain by the pre-frontal cortex. It's like changing the code on a computer. The computer (brain) obeys the instructions that the software (mind) gives it. With instant inductions, it's not exactly the same. Instant inductions work by pattern interruptions, not a progressive trance. For example, you might be familiar with the "Handshake Interruption" induction that a lot of stage hypnotists use. This is when you shake the hand of a member of your audience, then after your hand makes contact, you grab their extended arm with your other hand, interrupting the pattern. In that brief 1 to 3 second period where that pattern is confused, their brain is scrambling to figure out what is going on. It will then latch onto whatever you suggest as the answer to that confusion (as long as it doesn't violate their moral code). That's why they interrupt a pattern and say "Sleep!" and the person drops. You must set an expectation with your client for this to work. You cannot just pattern interrupt any random person and expect it to have the same effect. Just like progressive and rapid inductions, instant inductions work after your client agrees to be hypnotized. No one can be hypnotized against their will, and it would be unethical to even try to do that. I guess instant inductions could be done for hypnotherapy, but I have never really needed to do this. I guess I would if someone wanted to try it, but it's never been necessary. What is important to remember when doing progressive or rapid inductions is that your client does not need to be fully relaxed to be hypnotized. They also do not literally need to be asleep. The closest thing to actual sleep I've seen in a session is someone feeling somewhat unconscious for like 5 seconds but no more than that. Although very uncommon, even if someone forgot what you said during the session, this does NOT mean they were unaware or without control. Every person that is hypnotized is always 100% in control at all times. The reason you might say "Sleep" during an induction is that it helps to relax the client. Hypnosis as therapy is sort of like emulating sleep patterns without them being asleep. Dropping the biases of the pre-frontal cortex as if someone was asleep while keeping them awake. For progressive inductions, you first relax their body, then their mind. My personal favorite induction is called the "ceiling induction". In this induction, I have a person lay or sit down, then pick a spot on the ceiling. Then, I have them relax their whole body starting from the bottom of their feet, up to the top of their head, then forehead and face muscles. (You don't actually have to specify every muscle for them to relax. You could just say "Let your body relax.") Then I have them relax their mind and let it become open. After that, I have them go into a safe place and go from there depending on what they want to do. I don't want to go into every induction out there because there are many websites with thousands of scripts that you can read and study those inductions. You don't have to know every induction in order to be a hypnotist. It's more important to understand how the inductions work instead of memorizing lines from a script. If you understand the logic behind them, you can make an induction out of almost anything! The key is to not become a "follower" of any one hypnotist. Study from as many as possible and develop your own style. Another mistake people can make is to overdo the "relax" part of the session. You need to meet the client where they are. What would you do if someone has a lot of nervous energy and can't focus on your words? What if they feel stress when trying to be hypnotized? All thoughts and emotions can become a trance. You can turn the negative feelings into the solution which allows them to be hypnotized. For example: "I want to relax but I can't stop thinking about my job. I have a deadline I need to get done." In that case, I would say something like this. "That's okay. Actually, if you feel like you have to think about that deadline for now, then do that. You don't need to feel 100% relaxed to be hypnotized. Notice how the more you think about that deadline, the more you find it easier to relax. You don't have to stop thinking about that deadline if you don't want to. You can keep thinking about it if you want as you relax more and focus on the sound of my voice. If you want, you can let yourself keep thinking about it as you focus on the sound of my voice and relax deeper, or if you want, let that thought go immediately if that makes you feel better. Whether you hold onto that thought for now as you focus on the sound of my voice and go deeper, or you let it go completely and focus only on me, you can just relax now." You can do this with almost anything. The negative feeling is the trance (because they focus on the stress (focus) and it causes a behavior (being unable to focus)), so what you're actually doing is DE-HYPNOTIZING them by entering that trance and turning it to their advantage instead of a weakness. The goal is to turn all "issues" into strengths. Another way to do this is to say "That's okay, in fact, I don't know if you're going to stop overthinking now, in 5 seconds, 10 seconds, 15 seconds, or maybe minutes from now." One hypnotist had a client who felt the non-stop compulsion to argue with her husband. She realized this wasn't normal and wanted it to stop. When he was speaking to her on the phone, he said "I want you to hold onto this for now. Can you hold onto it until 9 PM? Don't let it go until 9 PM." She agreed, although somewhat confused by what he was saying. When she met up with him at his office, she explained to him that at EXACTLY 9 PM, she felt that compulsion vanish. Do you see what he did? By agreeing to hold onto it, she was actually agreeing to let it go. You can do this (indirect suggestion) for almost anything. This was a lifesaver for me. I had lifelong ADHD. For a lot of people, ADHD is tied to someone's mind trying to disassociate from stress. Basically, "I can't fix this, or run from this, so I'll disassociate to make myself feel better." (I don't know if this is true for everyone with ADHD. This is just my personal experience). So, anytime I had trouble focusing with my ADHD, I would just tell myself "That's okay brain, keep spacing out for another 5 seconds if you need to. Actually, don't stop doing that for 5, 10, or 15 seconds if you need to. The more you do that, the easier I find it to let it go." This always immediately gave me back my focus. The point being, if you say "I have XYZ problem and I need to fix it," then your mind is now actually molding it into a problem. It could be a problem OR a solution. Whatever suggestion you give to yourself is how your mind will take it. That's the beauty of self-hypnosis. You turn your issues into solutions. I now have a nearly unlimited attention span. This also applies to life situations. Say you made a bad financial decision. It's either "This was the worst decision I ever made. I shouldn't have done this. There is no way to fix this." Or, it's "I made a mistake, but making mistakes is experience. The more experience I have, the better financial decisions I'll make in the future and the wealthier I'll become." The things you say about your life experiences also act like suggestions. Either that traumatic experience was good for you because it made you wiser, or it destroyed you and you'll never come back from it. Your subconscious will accept whatever you decide to be the case, so choose well. Think of life as one big hypnotic experience. How will you hypnotize yourself? For better or worse? Nearly everything about your current life situation is the result of how you've decided to hypnotize yourself. You could say "That's not true! I can't control if the economy is bad! I can't choose how the market is going!" Sure, but there are people who PROFIT from a bad economy and people who LOSE from it. If you say that, you have decided that you are going to be the loser. If you say "The economy is bad, but that opens opportunities in other ways to make money," then your subconscious accepts the hypnotic suggestion you have given yourself and leads you to opportunities. Some people call this the law of attraction. Whether you believe there is a spiritual ability to manifest or not is your business. But, the more you realize that your life is in your control by your subconscious programming. Hypnosis can improve almost anything you can think of. People hypnotized for wealth will consciously and subconsciously be in a world of opportunity. People programmed for poverty will consciously and subconsciously always be in a world of lack.

CHAPTER FIVE:
HYPNOSIS FOR WEALTH & SUCCESS

Have you ever heard of "hypnotized for success" or "hypnotized for wealth"? How some people are "programmed for poverty"? What does this mean? It's very weird how people try to explain or advertise this as a service. "I can hypnotize you to be wealthy." Or "Manifest Wealth". How exactly do you "manifest" wealth? The reason is simple! Your subconscious mind will make you either successful or unsuccessful depending on the beliefs you have about money. Do you know how Nikola Tesla made his machines? He put himself into a trance and came up with an idea for an invention. Then, he asked his subconscious how to create the machine. His subconscious would then tell him step-by-step how to invent his idea down to the angle of the screws. You can do the same for success! If you say "It's hard to make money" then your subconscious accepts it, and you then subconsciously make decisions which make you poor. If you say "It's so easy to make money. What can I do next to make another $5000?" then your subconscious will respond in the same way it would answer Tesla. It will lead you to make decisions that make you wealthy! Do you know how to make 5 million dollars a year in real estate? Maybe not consciously, but your SUBCONSCIOUS knows exactly how to do this! So, by giving the subconscious positive instructions, you're actually leading yourself to the end goal. You "create" wealth the same way Nikola Tesla created his machines. One mistake is to develop an unnecessarily big ego. Dissolving your Ego is the key to success. Your bias might say that the best way to make money is to invest in cryptocurrency when the answer from the subconscious might be drop-shipping iPhone cables for $3 a piece off of Alibaba.com. It's the fact that "you," the conscious mind, doesn't know what to do that creates the success. You succeed by NOT knowing what to do! Because by being mentally open, you allow the subconscious to give you a much better answer than you'd get by having an Ego. This is also useful for salesmen and business owners. Most of my business ideas were given to me by my subconscious. A great way to supplement this is to expand your vocabulary. Learn what words mean. How can you turn something into an "asset" if you don't know the meaning of the word "asset"? Expanding your vocabulary allows you to come up with creative ideas for money-making. This is a very powerful tool to use. It lets you turn absolutely anything into a source of money. The subconscious only knows the present. When you present a clear, present-day statement combined with financial vocabulary, you allow the subconscious to fill in the gaps to make that statement your reality. Let's break down this statement: "My car is an asset". People usually think that asset means something you own. That is not true. An asset is something you own that MAKES YOU MONEY! If something you own costs you more money than it makes you, then it is a liability. My car IS an ASSET. You're stating to your subconscious that your car is CURRENTLY making you money. When you PRESENTLY state that something is an Asset and you understand the meaning of the word Asset, your mind now will flow with ideas on how to make that your reality. If your car is your asset, then how? Is it a commuter car you rent to people locally? Is it a luxury car you rent to rappers for their music videos? Do you rent it to celebrities? You can do this with literally anything. "This straw in my cup is an Asset." Say that, and your subconscious will give you the ideas to make that a reality. Do you sell straws? Do you sell the materials to make straws? Do you buy straws in bulk then sell them in smaller packs for larger profit? I've done this myself. As much as I love being a hypnotherapist, I ALSO love making money. Unfortunately, there are only so many people in every month who need to quit smoking, or lose weight. I've asked my own subconscious the question "How do I make six figures as a hypnotist." What was the answer for me? "Sell hypnosis tracks for an affordable price on the internet. Set up virtual sessions so you can find clients anywhere on earth. Run funny Ads on social media, and then find people who enjoy hypnosis enough that they would want retainer contracts." That is what has helped me earn a living in an incredibly unique and misunderstood field of work. Hypnosis for wealth and success also has to do with how someone feels about money. The things said to you about money from the time you were born can stay in your subconscious and manifest later as poverty. If you were told "Money is the root of all evil." or "Rich people are evil and greedy." then it can make you subconsciously avoid wealth like a sickness in an attempt to keep you safe. And, stop hating wealthy people! They're not all evil! It doesn't help that TV, Movies, Video Games, and many other media have made it look like all wealthy people are greedy. There are a lot of people who could be greedy while being rich. But, some wealthy people are just irritated with the public. Imagine that you came from nothing, and had to work your entire life for your success. Then, after all of that, you published books detailing EXACTLY how you did it so that other people could learn from your experiences and become successful too. Then, the majority of responses you got were people complaining that you're lazy, greedy, and selfish. That you're "one of the elites" as if you were somehow born into wealth. All the while they make absolutely zero effort to invest, trade, or even learn how money works! How would you feel? This is why a lot of wealthy people come off like they hate the poor. They don't actually hate poor people; they hate poor people who are lazy and have no interest in improving their life. Because the majority of those wealthy people had to struggle to get to the point that they are. You need to shift both your mindset and your relationship with money and wealthy people. Stop hating successful people, and learn from them instead. Shift your mindset from LOSER to WINNER! Money is NOT evil, and you should have as much of it as you can handle. Money allows you to provide for your family, help the needy, and pay for life-saving surgeries. Hypnosis for wealth involves you changing the relationship you have with money and setting specific goals. What does wealthy mean for you? 1 Million? 10 Million? Only hundreds of thousands? It also involves you reprogramming what you attract into your life. Your unconscious could incline you to take the door on the left, which leads to the room with credit card debt. It could also lead you to the door on the right with $5,000 in cash. You don't know what is behind the door until you walk in. When you hypnotize yourself for wealth, you're making it so that the subconscious makes you automatically inclined to recognize which door leads where. Let me give you a personal example: I once wanted to buy a Ford Ranger truck. I had trouble finding one, and the few in my area were very pricey. I put myself in a trance, and visualized exactly the truck I wanted. This was to convince my subconscious that I already had this truck. Then, I took a notepad and wrote out affirmations of gratitude for this truck. A few days later, after my shift at my then job, I had a sudden urge to buy a cup of coffee. After that, I passed by a street with a truck and a big "For Sale" sign. Guess what kind of truck it was? 1990 Ford Ranger, excellent condition, with only 100k miles. This is how the subconscious can manifest wealth. Your version of the "truck" could be a desired piece of real estate. The point is that your subconscious knows the way to put you towards any goal you may have; you just need to be able to set a clear intention and declare it in the present.

CHAPTER SIX: HYPNOSIS FOR WEIGHT LOSS

How can hypnosis help people lose weight? Let's be honest, there are endless reasons someone might be unable to lose weight. This is assuming they're exercising regularly and eating a healthy diet. The three most common reasons a person cannot lose weight are:

1.

They're over-stressed. Stress can steal energy from a person's metabolism (hence the weight gain) and immune system. Basically, their metabolism is low on fuel. All stress is basically the same mechanism. It's not different types of stress but different amounts. Stress in the brain is an outdated mechanism where the body takes energy away from its metabolism (and other functions of the body) and uses it to fight predators. The "stress" mode in the brain was only developed to be used temporarily, not for long periods of time. If you're constantly stressed, then your body is constantly in "fight mode" and steals energy away from your metabolism, which is why some people can't lose weight when they're eating healthy and exercising.

2.

They feel unloved. This doesn't really need much of an explanation. Sometimes when someone feels unloved, their body compensates by holding onto excessive weight.

3.

They have a subconscious belief that their metabolism is weak. This is usually just from suggestions they were given by their parents. It's more or less a feeling of inadequacy in their body. You see this in people with incredible metabolisms. They almost always tell you "I can eat ANYTHING and not get fat!". Self-suggestions and belief take a big part in this result. The subconscious uses the nervous system to communicate information to your body. If you believe your metabolism is weak and you give the command, then your body will obey that suggestion and follow suit. Whether it's stress, feeling unloved, their beliefs, or even something else, the way you approach it doesn't have to be that much different. It's better to not bring up each of these points, and instead let the answer come up as an insight from the person's subconscious. Avoid saying something like "It might be stress." while they're under hypnosis. If it isn't stress, you could then be adding to their list of reasons! It would be better to use an indirect or direct suggestion to reveal the answer from their subconscious while also removing the issue at hand. "You don't need to know why this **used to be a**n issue, but you could choose to know if you wanted to. If you want to walk through the door on the left, you'll remember why this **used to be** an issue for you, and you'll find it so much easier to just **let it go now** if you want... Or, you could take the door on the right, if you don't really need to know why it **was** a problem for you in the past and find it so easy to just let it go without having to remember why..." Like I mentioned before, the subconscious knows ONLY the present! They're not going to lose weight in the future, they've ALREADY lost the weight. They're ALREADY at the weight that they want to be. They're either CURRENTLY LOSING the weight or have ALREADY lost it! Do not say "You will lose weight in the FUTURE". This says that they have NOT lost the weight, and can actually roadblock the weight loss process because there IS NO future in the mind of the subconscious unless you set a specific date (For Example: At 1:40 PM on September 19th, I will lose 10 pounds).

It can help to approach the hypnosis at multiple angles. You could hypnotize them to eliminate stress, then have them imagine their new body (in the present) where they've lost that weight and feel so much more relaxed and at ease. Where the more they feel relaxed, and let go of the stress, the more they lose the excess weight. And, the more they lose excess weight, the more they feel relaxed, which creates a perfect cycle. First, try to do a general insight to find out why they can't lose weight, then adapt the suggestions to the answer they receive from their subconscious. Another way to do this is to bring them deep enough to have their subconscious speak and answer questions. If you do this, ALWAYS phrase the question as if the weight issue was in the past! "Why did Mark have trouble losing weight in the past?", "Work Anxiety".

CHAPTER SEVEN: HYPNOSIS FOR SLEEP ISSUES

Hypnosis works amazingly for people struggling with sleep-related issues. The most common that I have seen is usually insomnia, or waking up multiple times during their sleep cycle. Every case is different, but 99% of the time it's caused by a person worrying over something they don't realize they're worrying over. Anxiety can be subtle, and unnoticed. Many people have disassociated their anxiety to the point they don't really feel it, but it can still manifest in little ways like insomnia, or waking up while you sleep. Helping someone with this is kind of similar to weight loss hypnosis. Don't push to find out why they have the issue, but let it come up naturally. You don't always need to know why a client is having their problem, but if you delve into it, let it come up NATURALLY. Use direct / indirect suggestions intelligently to draw out the answer instead of forcing it. Having the subconscious answer a question is useful for a situation like this. One person I was working with kept waking up multiple times during the night. He had no idea why. It had been happening for about 3 to 4 months and for seemingly no reason. I hypnotized him, and asked his subconscious what was going on that was causing this to happen. It responded, "Work stress. He recently moved. It's him moving and his work stress." I then asked, "What does he need to feel better from this situation?" "Assurance," it responded. "What kind of assurance?" I asked it one last time. "Assurance that things will get better. That's what he needs." This showed that his "sleep issue" wasn't a sleep issue; it was anxiety. Instead of only focusing on his sleep, I had him imagine that as he worked his shift at his job, he was completely shielded from any and all negativity (visualization of a white light bubble) and that no matter what anyone else said or did, it didn't matter because that shield kept him safe at all times. Then, as he visualized himself in the third person watching himself sleep, any negativity was bounced away by this invisible shield. Another thing that I included was that every day he worked at his job, he found that he was moving closer to his goals. And no matter what his job entailed, it always pushed him closer to his dream life. I did 2 more reinforcement sessions after this, and it completely resolved his sleep situation. You need to meet people where they're at for this type of hypnosis.

Don't bring in your own Ego, and like I've mentioned before, let people's natural insights from their subconscious give the answers to why they are dealing with what they are having to deal with. Once their subconscious provides the reason, give suggestions that assist in that as well as have the person visualize themselves sleeping in the third person. Let them watch themselves sleeping soundly from the time they hit the bed to the time they wake up. The suggestion I gave my client was, "When you decide it's time to go to bed and you're laying on your bed, you find it easy to sleep soundly and quickly drift off and relax as you watch yourself in the third person fall asleep..." It's important to be very specific. Don't say "When you want to sleep, you find it easy to instantly fall asleep" Or, "When you are tired, you can instantly fall asleep." You don't want him to LITERALLY fall asleep anytime he gets tired. What if your client is a truck driver and gets tired while he's driving? Do you want him to instantly fall asleep then? That's why my suggestions were that he could quickly fall asleep when he wants to, in his room, and on his bed or couch. Be very careful how you word things. Generally, the subconscious wouldn't accept the suggestion in the wrong context, but it's not something you want to test. Also, check to see if your client has a medical diagnosis related to their sleep issue. If they have a diagnosis, it doesn't always mean that you can't work with them, but you need to have them ask their doctor to sign off saying they can get hypnosis. Doctors don't usually have an issue with hypnotherapy, so this doesn't really ever create a problem, but unless you are a licensed doctor in your state, it's what you need to do as a hypnotherapist. Consult with lawyers in your state to find the limits of what you can and cannot do as a hypnotherapist. I believe there is one state where only doctors can use the term "hypnotherapist," and that is New York. But, you can still be a "hypnotist" who does "hypnotism". A little bit strange, but that's because hypnotherapy is an unknown and uncommon work. It's not so much that doctors are "hiding it"; it's just not very common for them to learn in medical school. You don't want to come off like you're dismissing their practice as a doctor, only supplementing what they're doing with their patient. It's not your place to demean or dismiss any doctor's practice.

CHAPTER EIGHT: HYPNOSIS FOR PTSD AND ANXIETY

Hypnosis is an amazing tool for resolving PTSD. The truth is that VERY few people (especially people who treat PTSD) actually understand how PTSD works. They think it's simply just an overactive part of the brain (specifically the Amygdala, which deals with fear and stress). They misunderstand WHY the panic-attacks are so vivid and real to you when you're experiencing them. It's because your subconscious only knows the PRESENT and cannot distinguish reality from imagination. Do you remember when you were a child and would play pretend? If you imagined yourself climbing up a huge ice mountain, you would really feel like you were there! You'd feel the cold of the temperature on your skin, the weight of the snow as you'd walk up the mountain. You'd hear in your mind all the noises of the wind as it hit your face. It was so vivid you could feel all the sensations in your body as you'd pretend you were really there. Your subconscious can emulate sensations like temperature, emotions, sound, even hallucinations (common stage hypnosis trick) vividly as if it was really happening. You see a lot of this in stage hypnosis performances! People can be made to hallucinate, feel sensations, and hear things that aren't there. There are many false experiences that can be emulated by the subconscious. PTSD is like your subconscious is "playing pretend" with horrible memories! You know those relaxation exercises? They have you imagine yourself on a sunny beach, the sand on your feet, the sound of the ocean, the warmth of the sun? It can REALLY feel like you're there. Now, imagine the complete OPPOSITE of that! What if you were so immersed, but it was something horrible? The memory of sexual abuse, robbery, witnessing a murder, horrible military experience, or anything that traumatized you! This could create a false experience of sensation which would feel like it was real! It's similar to how a file is saved on your computer. Once a file (memory) is saved on your computer, you can open it and change the file or leave it be! If you have a text document on your computer that says "apples," it will not change to "oranges" until you open the file, re-write the text, and save it. Similarly, your brain has a catalog of memories. When the memories are replayed, they are experienced more or less the same as when it was registered. You can see this in people who recall memories from their childhood; they go from a mundane, monotone 45-year-old man with a wife, kids, and mortgage to that happy, excited 10-year-old who just got his first Nintendo. You'll see their face light up as they become EXACTLY who they were (in tone of voice and mannerisms) when that memory was registered. So, what about a scared, four-year-old kid who was sexually abused by his uncle? When that memory is replayed in their subconscious, they become that same helpless child. Part of the solution is to CHANGE the memory itself! Play pretend with it! It's basically your subconscious "playing pretend" with a memory, just like you could play pretend as a child (which is why PTSD memories are so vivid to begin with). YOU have the power to change the memory! YOU can use hypnosis to re-write that memory and change the ending! Will that change what happened? No! But, it can spare you all the panic attacks! For example: If you had PTSD from a car crash, and cars triggered the panic attacks, then what you could do is do hypnosis, recall UP UNTIL THE CRASH, and then CHANGE what happens! Once you CHANGE what happens, the subconscious responds to the NEW story of this memory and replays it how YOU want! Instead of the car crashing, a giant bubble enveloped it and floated it away from yours! Instead of the car crashing, your car activated its hover-rockets and flew right over it! Or, good thing your car was a super titanium steel TANK that has shock absorption, which means only THEIR car got damaged. Your car was so safe that it never even got a dent! You got shot? Is that your PTSD? Well, actually, when you got shot, bubbles came out! No, actually, you were wearing a bulletproof vest! Or, wait, guns aren't even real! So, who cares?! Generally, when you remember something, you remember it the way you LAST recalled it! So, once you recite the memory (under hypnosis) and you change the story and outcome, exiting the memory can "save the file" of the memory on your subconscious' database of memory. Also, many people might be "holding onto it" because there was no justice for what happened. It's anger. If you're doing hypnosis for someone in this situation, separate the anger and move it into its own category. Make their need for justice separate from their panic attacks and PTSD. Indirect suggestions are extremely useful for PTSD hypnosis. Some people do well with direct suggestions, but you want to approach it extremely relaxed. You want to be gentle with how you approach this. You're NOT having them relive this experience. In fact, they're (while in hypnosis) watching it from a TV screen! Use gentle, safe language when doing ANYTHING with PTSD. If anything, bring them up to the point where it happened and CHANGE the result QUICKLY! Don't let confusion linger, or panic can come out. If it was a car crash, then as soon as you get to the point where the crash happened, you IMMEDIATELY change the memory! Another way you can do this is to change what and who they are when this happened. If they were sexually abused as a child, then they are now an ADULT who can protect themselves instead of a small, defenseless child. Now, when their abuser comes into the room to harm them, they are now an ADULT with a gun at their side. CHANGE the STORY, and OUTCOME of the memory AS WELL as who they are! If you have them remember the memory while painting them as a defenseless child (or in a vulnerable position, say not wearing a bullet-proof vest when shot), then it can reinforce a negative part of the memory. They are now invulnerable to harm in this memory, and the outcome is that the ABUSER or THREAT is no longer in power! I do not recommend doing PTSD hypnosis if you're a beginner hypnotist who has no experience with this! Don't even touch it if you don't know what you're doing! But, if you're an experienced hypnotist (who has the legal permission from their doctor, as PTSD can be classified as a medical disorder and you are not a licensed physician) and you are working with someone who has PTSD, then I hope this can help you improve their experience during their session. If you're someone looking for a hypnotist to work with you on PTSD (If you are diagnosed with PTSD, otherwise it's just anxiety), then first get a note from your doctor authorizing you to get hypnotherapy, and either contact me (541-450-9722, elijah@alpha-hypnosis.com, alpha-hypnosis.com) or find a qualified hypnotherapist in your area and show this chapter to them! I hope to get this out to as many people as possible! Note, this is NOT meant to replace medical treatment or intended as medical advice. Always consult your doctor for medical advice and/or diagnosis. When you're doing hypnosis for anxiety, it's similar to hypnosis for PTSD, but you're really trying to identify WHAT they mean by anxiety. No matter what the issue you're dealing with is, you need to set a specific outcome. Are they trying to get rid of it completely? Have your client (if you're a hypnotist) explain to you EXACTLY what they want! Some want just a little bit of relief; others want total relief and to never be bothered by their anxiety at all. When you set a specific goal, you can have them visualize their ideal life under hypnosis and make it their present reality. Always make sure you understand what exactly they want, so you don't bring your own ego into it. What do they mean by anxiety? One person I helped described it as being angry around their children because they were low on energy. ALWAYS elaborate with a WHY! Why do you feel angry when they do this? "Because I am overwhelmed, and they got on my last nerve. They're taking away my peace and it pisses me off. I love them, but I want my time too!" Have them elaborate, and set their desired goal. Ok, so it's not just generic "anxiety"; it's being frustrated with not having enough me-time, and being overwhelmed. 90% of "anxiety" sessions are usually a DEEPER issue which you need to find out! If it's feeling overwhelmed, then one thing you could give as a suggestion is "Whenever you take care of your children, you're reminded of how temporary this situation is. The more your children grow up, the less immediate energy they'll take from you... as it makes you treasure the time you spend realizing they're only little for so long...". If it's anxiety that's really just anger, you could say, "You now realize that you're in control... Anytime you're in this situation, you now realize that no matter what they may do or how the situation might seem, you always feel in control and are confident it will always be this way...". You can also do something similar for PTSD hypnosis, "I understand you can feel angry (only say this if they have mentioned they are angry, don't bring in an additional problem!) but isn't your need for justice separate from anger? I won't say anger is bad... but isn't it better for you to be of a clear mind to get the best possible justice? If anger controls you, then maybe you are motivated to let it go as you're reminded that peace of mind brings the best possible justice..." You don't have to say this word for word but adapt it! Turn all WEAKNESSES into STRENGTHS! EVERY anxiety session is different! Find out the specific emotions they feel (fear, anger, overwhelm, fatigue) and ADAPT IT! Remember! Don't say that ANYTHING is a "problem", but rather a MISUSE of a tool! Anger, fear, hate, overwhelm, disgust, guilt (under the umbrella of "Anxiety") are all natural emotions. They aren't "problems" needing to be fixed, but tools that are misused! RE-FRAME their "issue" into a strength! Change HOW they feel XYZ emotion and WHAT triggers it; don't remove it as a problem. Indirect suggestions are extremely useful for dealing with anxiety-related issues! In fact, go a step beyond! Explain to your client how their mind isn't sick! They need more than just a hypnosis session; they need to understand that it's possible to re-frame their "issues". Make them walk out of that session feeling more in control than ever! As a hypnotist, your job isn't just to solve meager inconveniences but to empower people to live better lives! As much as I'd like to write multiple pages about this, there's really no need. It's basically what I just said: find a specific emotion behind their "anxiety", set a specific goal, re-frame don't "fix" (what isn't broken), and EMPOWER your clients!

CHAPTER NINE: PAST LIFE HYPNOSIS

I'm sure you've heard of "past life regression" hypnosis before. Now, what the hell are past lives? Well, honestly, as much as I'd like to just say the answer, I don't think it's my place to. I know, but there's the basic answer. Almost every living soul has had past lives, hypnosis can make someone remember past lives, and there is life after death. Some people are going to read that and dismiss that as bullshit, others will have an unquenchable thirst to find out the answer! If you really want to know, CONTACT ME (541-450-9722, elijah@alpha-hypnosis.com), and if you feel like it doesn't really matter, then feel free to skip this part of hypnosis! However, you do need to know that some health-related and psychological issues can be related to past lives. Sometimes it was an experience that happened 9 past lives ago. One thing to note, people's egos can create false identities for their past lives. Sure... 20 DIFFERENT PEOPLE were Ghengis Khan... If at any point you are working with someone and their subconscious tells you their issue is related to a past life, feel free to let it know that that time has passed, and that they, in their new identity and body, are safe. You also may hear your client's subconscious mention something called a "higher self" and that you can speak to it. I'll probably write a different book for what all of this means, but if this happens, it can be useful to speak to this "higher self", and if you do, then ask it what message it has for your client. I can do past-life regressions, but I don't really advertise as a "Spiritual Hypnotist". As obvious as it is that there is the existence of a spiritual realm, and spirits in this world... some people believe we're only evolved primates and we have no soul. I respect everyone's beliefs, but if you have a belief system like this, you might find yourself stumbled in your journey to taking back your control.

CLOSING CHAPTER: THANK YOU FOR READING!

Thank you for reading this book! I hope to get this out to as many people as possible! If you have any questions, don't hesitate to contact me through my social media, or my information (541-450-9722, ELIJAH@ALPHA-HYPNOSIS.COM (mailto:ELIJAH@ALPHA-HYPNOSIS.COM), alpha-hypnosis.com). If you're just interested in hypnosis and how it can help you, I offer free sample sessions for anyone wanting to try it! Contact me to see if it's for you! If you're interested in becoming a hypnotist, then I hope you'll find the information in this book useful on your journey! I actually have a group of hypnotists who help people looking to get into it. You can join this group on my website alpha-hypnosis.com. It's absolutely free, no ranks or fees, and everyone is welcome. I plan on make more books about hypnotherapy, but I wanted to make one explaining the basic. Don't try to learn everything at once, test the waters until you find your way!

www.ingramcontent.com/pod-product-compliance
Lightning Source LLC
Chambersburg PA
CBHW071000220526
45471CB00007B/3114